# Yoga and Your Mental, Spiritual and Physical Health

**An Introduction to Yoga and Its Many Uses**

By: Aileen Gomez

9781681275239

# PUBLISHERS NOTES

## Disclaimer – Speedy Publishing LLC

This publication is intended to provide helpful and informative material. It is not intended to diagnose, treat, cure, or prevent any health problem or condition, nor is intended to replace the advice of a physician. No action should be taken solely on the contents of this book. Always consult your physician or qualified health-care professional on any matters regarding your health and before adopting any suggestions in this book or drawing inferences from it.

The author and publisher specifically disclaim all responsibility for any liability, loss or risk, personal or otherwise, which is incurred as a consequence, directly or indirectly, from the use or application of any contents of this book.

Any and all product names referenced within this book are the trademarks of their respective owners. None of these owners have sponsored, authorized, endorsed, or approved this book.

Always read all information provided by the manufacturers' product labels before using their products. The author and publisher are not responsible for claims made by manufacturers.

*This book was originally printed before 2014. This is an adapted reprint by Speedy Publishing LLC with newly updated content designed to help readers with much more accurate and timely information and data.*

Speedy Publishing LLC

40 E Main Street, Newark, Delaware, 19711

Contact Us: 1-888-248-4521

Website: http://www.speedypublishing.co

REPRINTED Paperback Edition: 9781681275239:

Manufactured in the United States of America

# Dedication

This book is dedicated to my yoga partner, Lyn. Thank you for patiently waiting for me every day so we can do yoga together.

# TABLE OF CONTENTS

# CHAPTER 1- THE THREE PILLARS OF YOGA

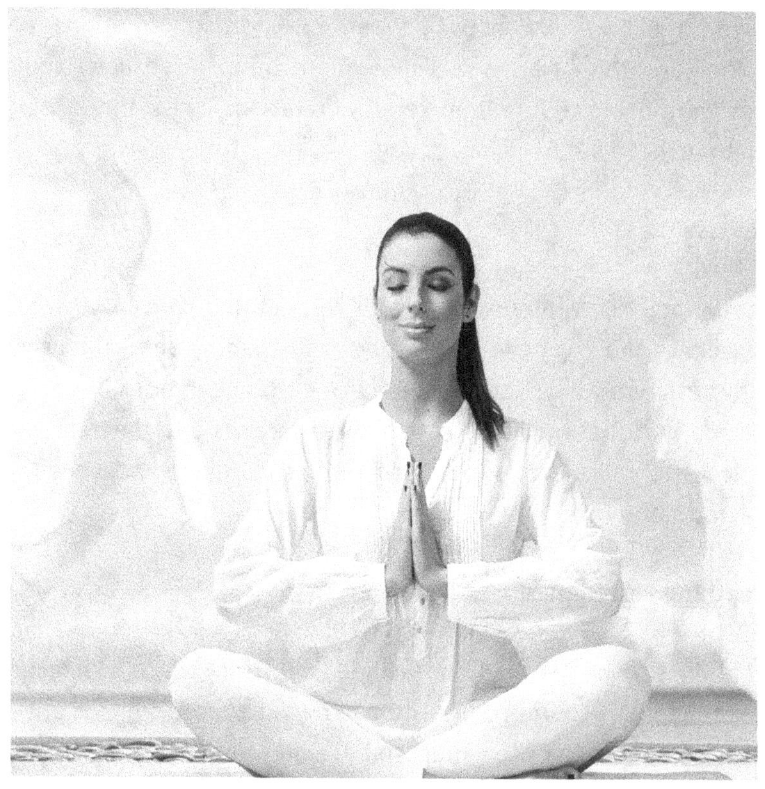

Yoga is basically an ancient knowledge of body which originated from Indians and it is more than 500 years old. The basic word of yoga is originated from a Sanskrit word "yuj" which means to unite or to integrate two things. Yoga is exercised and practiced to unite your body with your spirit or you can make it easier and say that the reunion of person's own consciousness and universal consciousness is achieved through yoga.

Ancient people, who practiced yoga, believed in the fact that in order to achieve internal peace, a person must integrate and unite his mind, body and spirit. Without this reunion, person can never achieve internal peace.

This is very dense and difficult process to unite all three of the above because you need extraordinary control over your emotions, intelligence and actions. Yugis developed some easy and short cut ways to achieve balance between intelligence, emotions and actions and this balance was dependent upon three basic things that were exercise, breathing and meditation. These three things are thought to be the pillars of yoga.

**Exercise**

Human body is treated with lots of respect and care in yoga and this allows the yoga exercises to be very friendly and calming for body structure. Once you start practicing these exercises, then, you will see that there is no twist in these exercises and they are very basic poses which are formulated by yogis to develop peace within the body structure.

**Breathing Techniques**

Breathing techniques were included in this process because breathing is the source of life and when your source of life is out of order then, how can you expect to have harmony and order in your life.

Breathing techniques help person to gain control over his whole body and his whole internal system as well. These techniques are little difficult to learn but yoga is all about practice and you can learn them by regular practice easily.

**Meditation Techniques**

Meditation is another thing which is necessary for yoga practice but there is some misconception involved about this technique and people think that their mind has to go blank for meditation.

This is not the case because meditation is just another self-controlling technique which allows you to think more clearly and it harmonizes your thoughts and actions. All three of the above things are very necessary part of yoga and you have to learn all three of the above step by step. You can say these techniques are the stairs to master yoga.

Most of the people become hesitant and say that they have never done any stretching exercise and they cannot learn the difficult poses of yoga but this is a wrong thinking. Yoga is for everyone who wants peace and harmony in his life. There is nothing in this world which is made and designed for specific people instead all humans have equal capabilities and everyone can practice and master yoga.

You just need to concentrate very hard on these skills and integrate them in your life in such a way that they become your habit. There is a saying that you should make yoga so much important part of your life that you may forget to eat but you should never forget to practice yoga.

This saying can tell you the importance of regularity in yoga. The first thing which yoga will give you will be a great looking and perfectly healthy body which everyone wants and after that later stages of breathing techniques and meditation appear.

**Possible Side Effects of Yoga**

As with most things, Yoga has side effects if one does not take the time to understand the endeavor embarked upon. Yoga is no different, though it is known for its grace and gentleness, it should be taken for granted and certainly should be deviated until and unless one understands the possible consequences of the deviation.

Some yoga movements consist of really hard to do maneuvers though it may look easy to start with, therefore it is very important to start the yoga adventure under supervision of an experiences yoga practitioner. If wrongly executed, these poses can result in serious injury or simply be useless in terms of what the individual is trying to get from it.

Consulting a physician is also a good idea before thinking of embarking on any yoga program. Some people do so without this vital doctor's input and even wrongfully decide not to continue with the ongoing treatments and medications and replace it with yoga. This elimination is only advised and possible when some positive results are forthcoming.

Besides experiencing pain in the wrist, neck, and back areas, some people have experienced ligament tears and tendons and muscles pull. There are even cases recorded stating the side effects of vertigo though this is indeed rare. There have also been cases of gastric problems that may occur upon commencing a yoga series of classes.

One of the possible explanations given for this gastric condition is that the given set of poses is not executed in the proper sequence and thus causing the discomfort. There are also instances of nausea, sour stomach, and vomiting.

When the yoga exercise is taken too seriously and the warning signs of discomfort are ignored and allowed to continue unaddressed, then some frighteningly serious consequences may occur such as internal bleeding, severe muscle strains, and ruptures. In these cases immediate medical helps needs to be sought.

# CHAPTER 2- THE 6 BRANCHES OF YOGA

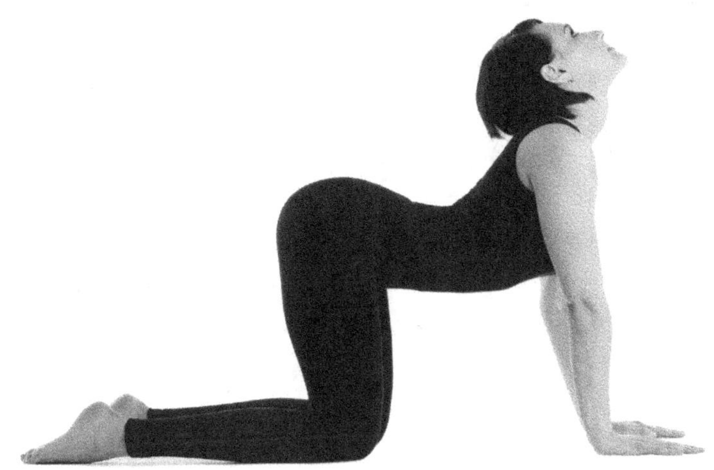

As I mentioned above that Yoga was originated from Indians and it is a very ancient art with lots of skills and complexities involved. If you think that yoga is just about posing your body in difficult positions then, you are mistaken because there are different branches of yoga which are listed below.

**Hatha Yoga**

Hatha yoga is also called yoga of postures and it is most famous branch of yoga in west which you must have seen. In this branch, body is twisted in different difficult and easy postures. The basic emphasis of this branch is to achieve peace through physical exercises, breathing techniques and mediation. Basic purpose of this yoga branch is to achieve better health along with spirituality.

This is the easiest branch as well because it does not take too much time from your busy routine and you can learn and master this art along with your daily work. You can easily adjust your schedule to practice and your daily routine will not be disturbed with this yoga branch.

## Bhakti Yoga

Bhakti yoga is not very popular in the west but it is most practiced branch of yoga in India. This involved spirituality more than physical gestures and it revolves around heart and divine. You have to choose a path which suits your hear desires most and then, you have to see everything and everyone through that path. Bhakti yoga allows you to develop your faith in something and they take that faith to that level where it can tell you the exact way to catch.

## Raja Yoga

Raja yoga is also called yoga of self-control. Even though self-control is characteristic of almost every yoga branch but this branch pays special attention to self-control. Most of the people who practice this branch of yoga are members of some religious prestige. Raja yogi sees him as central and gives respect to everything around.

The basic step in mastering self-control is to allow you to be discovered. Discipline learning is the basic characteristic of raja yoga and if your life is distracted and undisciplined then, you must practice raja yoga to gain control of your life and make it more disciplined.

## Jnana Yoga or Yoga of Mind

Jnana yoga which is also called yoga of mind deals primarily with human brain and it tends to control the intelligence of people. In this yoga people learn to integrate wisdom and intellect and with combination of these two, they try to create a perfect moment in their life when they never make wrong decisions. People who practice jnana yoga are very open minded and they keep learning about other religions, professionals, in order to expand their knowledge as they believe that expanding the knowledge expands their mental and intellect strength.

**Karma Yoga**

Karma yoga believes that you can make your future better by doing kind and selfless deeds in the present. It also believes that if your present is uncertain and hard then, it is the result of your past deeds.

Yogis, who practice karma yoga, do selfless help of other people, in order to make sure that their kindness to other people will make their future a better place. Karma yoga changes their whole concept of good and evil which changes their internal soul and makes them a better person with a bright destiny.

**Tantra Yoga**

Tantra yoga is the yoga of rituals but most of the times; it is misunderstood by many people because they rename it as sex yoga. Sex is just another part of this yoga but this is not all about tantra yoga. Yogis who practice tantra yoga possess certain qualities like purity, humility, devotion, dedication to his Guru, cosmic love and some others.

These are all the branches of yoga but there are some misconceptions also there about yoga for example some people say yoga is a religion but it is not. Yoga is just a way to make your life better and integrate peace in your life. It helps you to achieve a better life with more control over your mind, thoughts and actions. Yoga is also taken as just an exercise to keep your body fit which is true to some extent but it is not the whole concept of yoga. Exercise and physical health is just small portion of yoga but the higher aim of yoga is lot more sacred and important.

**What is Hot Yoga?**

Like its title this form of yoga is predominantly practiced in hot and humid surroundings which have this constant temperature atmosphere.

Apparently there are other effects that can occur with this particular feature incorporated into the sessions of yoga. It is interesting to note that though yoga is a very gentle and slow moving art form, the individual can complete the session not only feeling rejuvenated but also a little sweaty. Therefore when the hot yoga style is practiced there is also the aim in mind to really sweat out the unwanted negative elements of the body. None of those who use this style find the excessive perspiration an unpleasant byproduct, in fact most welcome it.

Hot yoga is a set series of yoga poses specifically designed to be carried out in a hot or heated room. In most cases the temperature of the environment where the hot yoga is done is kept at about 95 – 100 degrees. By mere virtue of the temperature alone the level of perspiration is quite high, coupled with the yoga exercises, the body is able to harness and emit a different level of warmth which in turn is purported to make the individual's body more supple and flexible.

The following are some of the benefits derived from the hot yoga style:

• The body's ability to burn fat is heightened

- The fluidity of the joints, muscles, ligaments and other supporting structures of the body are enhanced.

- Tissues and muscles are more effectively oxygenated because the capillaries better dilate with the heated surroundings.

- Peripheral circulation improves due to the enhancement of sweating.

- The metabolism rate speeds up

- The cardiovascular system gets a more strenuous work out though it is kept at a comfortable level

- The sweating element provides the detoxification and elimination of toxics through the skin.

# Chapter 3- How to Start Practicing Yoga

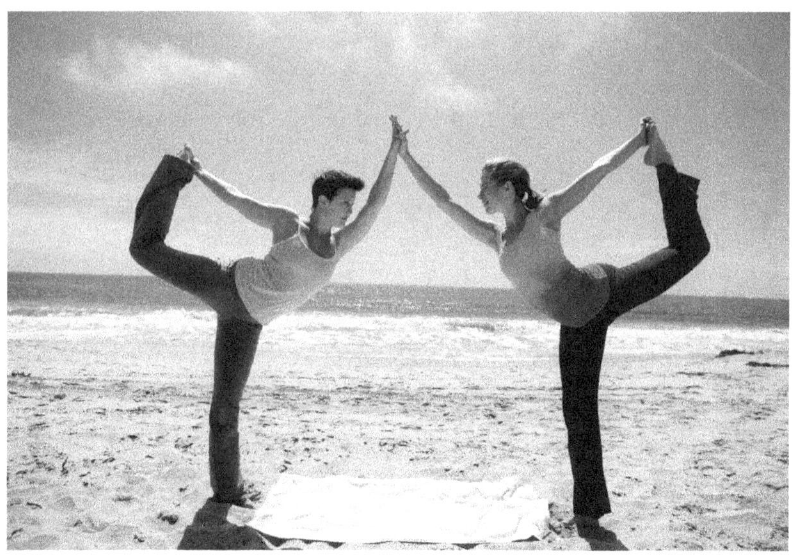

If you are planning to start practice of yoga then, you must know about certain things and in fact if you say more precisely then, there are 6 major things which you must know. These things are listed below and read them carefully for proper implementation of yoga exercises and techniques.

**Check Your Physical Health Status**

This is basic thing to know about your physical ability. Though the starting work of yoga will not be very tough and anyone can execute it perfectly but as the time passes and you advanced in these techniques, these will keep becoming tougher.

In order to adopt yoga properly, you should have your physical checkup before starting yoga and make sure that you do not execute any techniques which your body does not allow you to do. In this physical checkup, if you find out that you have certain disorder or weakness in some muscle then, you can change your routine accordingly.

## Concentrate On Just Yourself

When you join certain yoga learning classes then, you will come across wide range of people and some of them will be way ahead of you in practicing yoga but this should not discourage you from your cause instead, take these classes as personal development area where everyone is responsible for him or herself.

If someone is ahead of you then, this means he or she has practiced more than you and not because he or she is better than you. So concentrate on just yourself and make sure that you are on the right path.

## Make Your Mind for Physical As Well As Mental Exercises

Some people have this misconception that yoga is all about physical exercise but this is not entirely true because yoga is about practicing mental exercises as well. You will always have to prepare yourself for that and believe in the fact that yoga is about 50 percent physical and 50 percent mental stamina. It is to create a harmony between your mind and your body. This harmony will need some struggle and hard work to be achieved.

## Choosing Appropriate Yoga Class

There are different techniques available for executing in yoga and you need to select one which suits your mood. There are techniques like breathing techniques, mental exercises and even in some cases, laughing is also used to increase strength.

You should do your research about all these techniques and select the one which you think is most interesting for you and you will do it from your heart. Never choose your yoga technique by looking at your friend because he or she may have different interest and this can lead to discouragement.

**Commitment is Necessary**

Commitment is very necessary in yoga like any other exercise plan because if you keep on changing the technique or you keep missing the classes then, it will disturb the whole schedule and instead of giving you relief and relaxation, this may lead you to unbalanced physical level which can be dangerous. In order to gather most advantage out of yoga, you need to be very consistent about your approach.

**Try To Find Pleasure and Fun in Yoga Classes**

This is most crucial thing for making your yoga practice very fruitful and effective that you need to enjoy your yoga classes instead of taking them as burden and forcing yourself to go down and practice, you should have a fun attitude and you should wait for these classes to start throughout the day. This approach can change the whole effect of yoga practice and you can see the results by adopting this approach.

# Chapter 4- Yoga Poses for the First-Timers

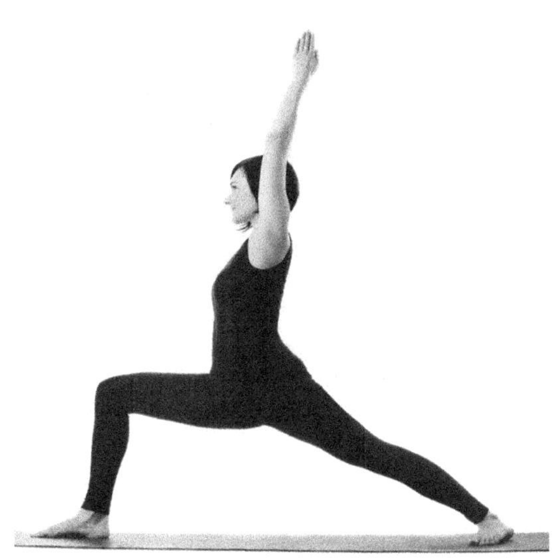

Hathe yoga which is also called yoga of poses is very famous in the west. Here are some of the basic and also some advanced poses which are exercised in yoga. Before learning these poses, you should learn some safety tips as well because if you exercised these poses in wrong way then, your body will get twisted and you may get hurt as a result.

• You need to be focused while practicing these moves and never think about anything else other that the move.

• Gentle approach should be applied because purpose of these moves is to gain comfort.

• Do not lose concentration and keep practicing.

• Try to observe the poses from pictures and try to perfect your angels.

**Basics of Yoga**

There are three things which are basic ingredients for learning yoga and these three things are breathing, movement and focus. If you can master and control these three things then, you will be able to learn yoga very fast. Deep breathing is the key and more deeply you breathe, more oxygen you will provide to your muscles and they will be able to adopt the technique.

Holding to these difficult poses need a strong body and physical health. You need to be very fit to exercise these poses effectively. You need to make your body very flexible to adopt difficult angels easily. Focus will give you enough power to harmonize both breathing and movement which will create an inner peace for you.

**The Candles Pose**

In this pose, you have to kneel on your shines and sit on your heels. Pressing your palms and heels together in front of your chest and taking a deep breath is the exact way to do it. You can repeat this pose 3-4 times easily.

**Mouse Pose**

Kneeling on your shines and sitting back on your heels is start of this pose. Bring chest close to your thighs and let your forehead rest on the floor. Stretch your arms behind you and let them relax. Relax all of your muscles and lay down in same position for some time. This is basically muscle relaxing pose.

**Dog Pose**

This is an advanced pose which starts from standing on both your arms and legs. Curl your toes and list your hips straight towards ceiling. In this position, you should look like in a V opposition. Your head should be hanging down to observe your own legs. You can learn this by watching a dog stretching after a nap. This pose allows you to strength all of your bones and muscles equally.

**Cobra Pose**

Lay down on your tummy with your legs straight. Place your arm on either sides and try to lift your chest as high as possible without moving your legs from straight position. Keep the shoulders wide and with an open chest, try to lift it even higher by pressing your hands on the floor. Your head should be straight with the shoulders and this pose can help you to relax your chest muscles as well as shoulders.

**Peacock Pose**

Sit up tall by widening your legs as wide as possible. Placing hands in front of you and pressing them to widen your shoulders will get you in this pose. This pose is little difficult to adopt but try and hold it for 5 deep breaths.

**Mountain Pose**

Stand straight up with your feet very close to each other. Bend your neck and look straight up in the ceiling. Let your arms relax on either sides and try to lift your chest. In this position, your head, shoulders and hips should be aligned. This pose is easier and you can hold this pose for 5-10 deep breaths.

**Butterfly Pose**

Sit by keeping the soles of your feet together. Rest your hands on your shoulders and lift and spread elbows wide. Flap your arms and legs gently like butterfly. You can repeat this process 15-20 times easily.

**Birds Pose**

In standing position, get your arms behind you and try to lift yourself on toe end of your feet. Be careful because most of the people fall while attempting this posture and you should rise up as much as you can and as soon as you start to lose balance, stop in that position and hold that position for 3-5 deep breaths.

**Fish Pose**

Lie down on the floor with your legs straight. Place your elbows on either sides and lift your chest with help of elbows as high as you can. Head should be very still and should rest on the floor. This is also a difficult pose and you should hold it for not more than 3 deep breaths.

**Do Nothing Doll**

Lie on your back in normal position and your arms open and palms facing skies. This is a total relaxing position and normally it is practiced at the end of all poses. Just close your eyes in this pose and try to relax. Think of yourself as a doll which has nothing to move. Stay in this pose for 5-8 minutes in the end of your yoga session.

# CHAPTER 5- ADVANCED YOGA POSES

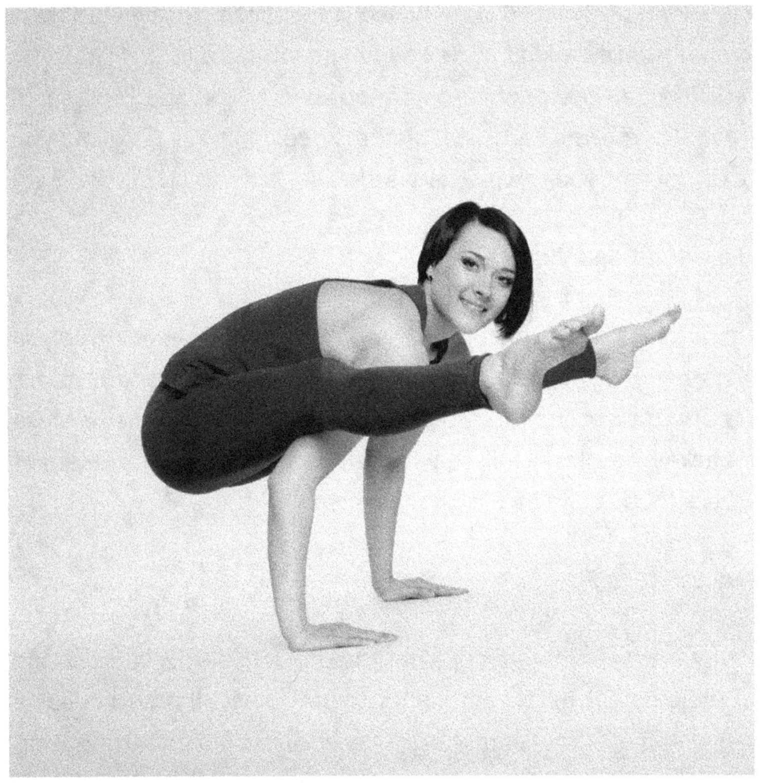

Once you have progressed from beginner's level to a higher level then, you need to change your poses and exercise some advanced poses because these poses will be more effective on you and you will not feel any trouble in implementing these advanced poses.

**The Bridge Yoga Pose**

This pose is a difficult pose and it is practiced when you are coming out of shoulder pose. To execute this pose perfectly, you need a very strong spine. If you are weak from your back then, you do not need to execute this pose as it can hurt your back.

**The Plough Yoga Pose**

This is another advanced pose which is for those people who have developed supreme kind of flexibility and strength in their muscles by practicing all the other ordinary poses of yoga. You can search internet and you will find exact pictures depicting this pose and you can execute it at your own after wards.

**The Forward Bend Yoga Pose**

This is another very difficult pose and in order to execute it you need to hold the toe ends of your feet for several deep breaths. This is also dangerous for people with any back problems because your back will suffer a full bend and if you have slight problem in your back then, it will invoke that problem.

**The Locust Yoga Pose**

This is another very tough pose but the difficulty is not in executing it but in holding it for several minutes and as usual, it also needs a very strong back. You should practice on basic poses and develop your back muscles to execute these poses effectively.

**The Bow Yoga Pose**

This yoga pose is just for expert yogis because it is difficult to execute and even more difficult to hold. You need tons of stamina and back strength which comes from years of practice. If someone challenges you to execute this pose then, you should think twice before accepting the challenge.

*Aileen Gomez*
## The Half Spinal Twist Yoga Pose

As it is evident from the name that it requires your spine to get twisted and to twist your spine, you need a back like rock which should never bother you in any position.

These are some of the yoga poses which are very difficult to execute and if you have noticed something that all of the above mentioned poses require very strong back.

They involve your back in the process somehow which demands that you should practice on regular and easy poses and develop your back so much that you can execute these advanced poses of yoga.

## Doing Yoga from Home

If you have learned yoga and you want to practice now at home without bothering about going in classes then, you must have some essentials at home which will help you in executing your yoga techniques more effectively and more properly.

## Choosing the Right Yoga Matt

Matt is the first essential thing which you must have in home and there are certain qualities of good quality yoga matt. First of all it should be very comfortable and smooth.

Thickness of matt also increases the comfort level but it will also increase the cost of matt. You can go with a medium thick matt for proper and healthy yoga practice.

You also should think about the cleaning method of your matt because if you are involved in hot yoga exercises then, matt will definitely get wet and will need to be washed. So look for a matt which you can wash in your washing machine easily.

**Other Miscellaneous Yoga Essentials**

Other than yoga matt, you should also carry a yoga bag and this is important because I have seen people who practice yoga that they do not care about their matt and towel and other things but you should have a proper bag which can hold all of your yoga items properly because discipline is first step of yoga and if you are not disciplined even in execution of yoga then, how can you expect any discipline in your life through yoga.

Some people will think that these essentials will cost them lots of money but believe it or not but all of the above items will not cost you more than $150. This is not a bog price to pay for proper execution of yoga in comfort of your house. So buy these accessories and exercise yoga at your home effectively.

# Chapter 6 - Yoga as Remedy to the Ailments of the Body

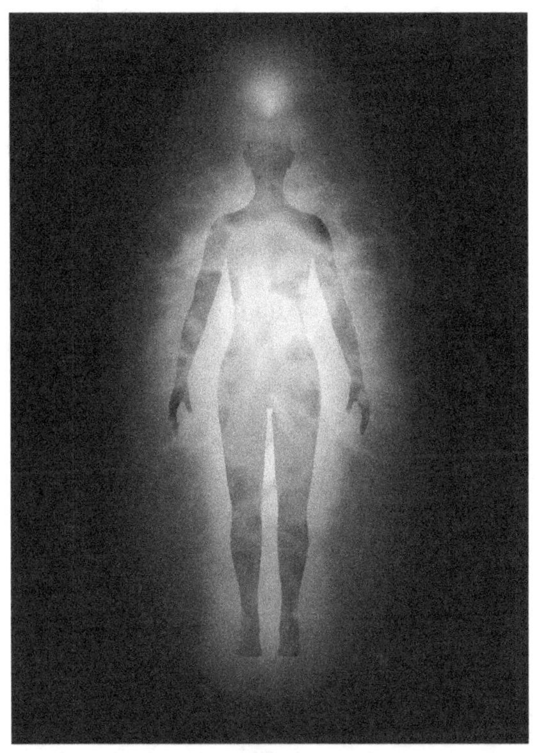

Yoga is taken as a physical remedy for many problems and especially for people, who tend to suffer from different health related problems like pain, stress, fatigue, sleeping disorder and other similar issues, yoga is perfect solution. It just needs a bit of practice and patience to see the results and initially, you can face some problems but as the time passes, you will learn the art of doing exercises properly and will start to relax after doing them. Following are the few advantages which you can get from yoga exercises.

**Increasing Flexibility**

Getting a flexible body is dream of almost every person but it is very tough to attain certain level of flexibility without proper exercise routine. All the exercises of yoga are based to increase stamina, flexibility and length of your muscles. I have seen people who started yoga when they were not even able to touch their foot toes but after some practice, they were able to bend their back completely without any trouble to touch their toes. Not only this but if you observe different poses of yoga then, you will know that it emphasis on certain parts of body which are almost ignored in daily routine but yoga exercises get these parts activated and makes them flexible to work.

**Increased Use of Joints, Ligaments and Tendons**

As I mentioned above that yoga increases flexibility and it is because of that long research of yoga positions. Every position is well-thought and well-conceived that you can activate your those parts of the body which are normally ignored for example, shoulder are a part of our body which can change our whole posture but we seldom do any exercise or certain movement which involved shoulders. In yoga, on the other hand, there are special postures which give stress and relax shoulder particularly and ultimately you make your shoulders strong and flexible.

**Increased Strength and Weight Management**

Yoga exercises help you in increasing the overall strength of all your body parts including your bones. This increased strength increases support for your whole skeleton. This is a great way to achieve a healthy and toned body. It not only increases the overall strength of your body but it also helps you in maintain your weigh because you have to practice different postures every day and in those postures, if your weight increases, you will notice it in very timely manner.

## Improved Blood Circulation

Yoga is recommended for patients who have increased blood pressure or even low blood pressure. There are different poses and exercises for both of these purposes. It regulates blood in a more proper way because the positions which are practiced in yoga are very precise and these positions make sure that every organ of the body comes in exact position which makes the job for the heat easier. It circulates the blood more easily and more properly.

## Detoxification

In yoga, muscles are stretched very gently and in some techniques massage are done and these techniques ensure proper blood flow in whole body which also works as detoxification of body. All the undesired secretions are effectively removes from the body because everything works in order.

## Stress Relief and Pain Relief

Cortisol is a substance in our body which controls the amount of stress and it is seen that all the yoga exercises help to reduce the amount of cortisol in human body which ultimately limits the effects of stress on our body. In ancient times, yoga exercises were used to cure different kinds of pain and in some parts of the world, some expert yogis still practice this technique of lowing and getting rid of pains.

**Focus On Present and Inner Peace**

Inner peace is a thing which is very rare in this materialistic world and through practice of yoga you can get this rare quality in yourself. Along with physical health, improving mental health is also a future of yoga exercises because it creates a harmony between thoughts, mind and actions of our body. It allows you to converge and focus your thoughts on one purpose of your life. It avoids all the distractions and enables your mind to think very clearly about the success.

**Yoga is Beneficial for All Age Groups**

If you observe yoga techniques then, you will notice that these techniques are not specific for any age group because some of these are very easy and some of them are complex which shows that people from any age group can practice these techniques and get results. In fact, as you keep on getting older, you master the art of yoga and all the skilled and prominent masters of yoga are very old aged people who have got all the control over these techniques and they are now teaching these techniques to their ancestors. Stamina increases with practice and people who have been practicing these techniques from young ages can become master of these arts in their older age.

**Better Breathing and Body Awareness**

When you keep on practicing yoga for longer periods of time then, you get a sense of awareness about your body and you know exactly what is going on inside your body. This helps you in identifying any faults and disorders very early in stage which helps to get rid of that disorder early.

With better breathing techniques, you feel comfortable and there are techniques in yoga which can enable you to attain relaxation in minutes. These techniques do not require any particular environment or timing and you can execute them even in your office chair to relax yourself.

## Helping Patients with Arthritis

Dealing with the arthritis condition can be very stressful and painful. Most arthritis sufferers diligently seek medical healing or alternative healing to help deal with the possibly debilitating disease. For most the recommendation given is couple a good exercise regimen with the necessary supplementation of other medical prescriptions. For those who have ventured into taking up yoga, have found that they managed to achieve wonderful percentages of recuperation, from this arthritis disease. Thus yoga has over time become the mainstream methods for dealing with arthritis conditions.

Yoga provides the gentle exercise routine for the arthritis patient who already has to endure the perpetual discomfort of pain. Each yoga move has a corresponding counter move and this helps to address the various muscles and joints which are affected by the arthritis condition. Many people who have tried yoga have attested to the almost immediate pain relief they have experienced after only a few supervised sessions.

When yoga is used as a form of treatment to address arthritis, the genes in the body which function as protector of pain and discomfort can actually be mare to function more efficiently to create a relaxed effect. This then allows the patient to find some immediate relief from the pain aspect produced from arthritis. Some researchers have linked arthritis to deep seated resentment building up in the individual's system. Thus with the help of yoga the deep seated resentment can be addressed by focusing on restoring the balance in the chakra system.

This chakra system is the primary energy vortex located along the spinal column and is associated with the energy of compassion and love for self and others. Yoga then helps to facilitate the means for the body to be rid of this negative energy pattern that is causing the arthritis disease, starting from the deepest levels.

**No More Painkillers for Chronic Back Pain**

Oftentimes people resort to pain killers or other medically prescribed items to control or reduce back pains. If the individual decides to try the art form of yoga to address back pain all these foreign substances can be avoided. Yoga is natural and does not have any of the possible side effects the prescribed medications may have. If done correctly, yoga can heal back pains effectively because of the stretching and exercising of both the muscles and joints. All it takes is a little yoga exercises every day. Once the positions most suited to the individual are narrowed down to address back pains, the movements can be practiced anytime.

In order to correct any back problems certain contributing factors need to be looked into. The incorrect posture, improper movements, or bad body mechanics, repetitive strenuous motions on the joints and muscles, disc injuries, damaged or inflamed ligaments are just some of these issues. With the correct supervised combinations of yoga movements all the above can be corrected, some gradually while others more quickly. Through the various yoga poses, specific areas of muscles and joints can be addresses and realigned to restore the centered positions in the body.

Some of the common positions that yoga uses to address the back pains are the locust pose, the cobra pose, and a few poses from the tadasasna regiment. Besides doing all the various yoga poses to enhance the back muscles and strengthen the posture, keeping other regular exercises as part of the daily routine is also recommended.

Simple exercises like swimming and light weight training are good ways to build and strengthen the back area. With the advancement of age, an individual should also be conscious of the strain on the back when lifting heavy objects or doing physically exerting exercises or work.

# Chapter 7- Calming Down ADHD and Emotions with Yoga

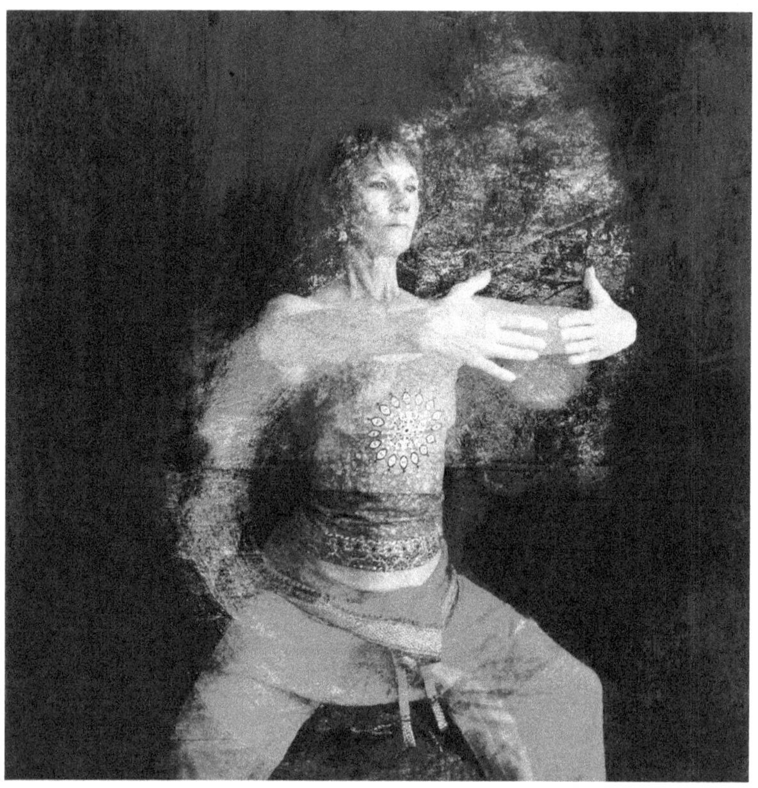

Yoga is an increasingly popular exercise module across the world. Since yoga can be performed in a small space, and gym membership is not necessary, its popularity has and will continue to grow. Beyond the convenience benefits yoga offers, regular participation has effects on both the body and mind. Yoga combines exercise with meditation, making it a manifold effort in controlling more than one area of need.

Yoga is another way to help individual with hyper activity problems. As this art form teaches the individual to increase the concentration levels and promotes mental and physical discipline it creates elements of confidence and the ability to focus better.

Balance is a technique practiced often in yoga exercises. Many of the positions involve shifting your weight to different parts of the body and balancing while breathing deeply. Controlled breathing exercises are associated with emotional management, which helps restore oxygen to the brain. All this further trains the individual to slow down and be focused.

In hyperactivity the link between the mind and body is disturbed, therefore with yoga the mind becomes more disciplined, while constantly promoting self-awareness and control. Yoga works to relieve the stress levels which are a further contributing factor for the individual who already has to deal with hyperactivity. Yoga improves the individual's ability to synchronize, de-stimulate an over active nervous system.

Another effect yoga can have when done on a regular basis is that it promotes strength, creating a stronger, leaner muscle. Exercises that build strength also promote sleep, which can help to regulate unhealthy sleep habits. Without enough sleep the problem-solving processes in the brain become diminished, which is another way yoga helps the mind to be able to operate at a high level. Yoga also improves concentration and creativity and creates sense of well-being and calm.

# Chapter 8- Yoga as Tool for Spiritual and Emotional Healing

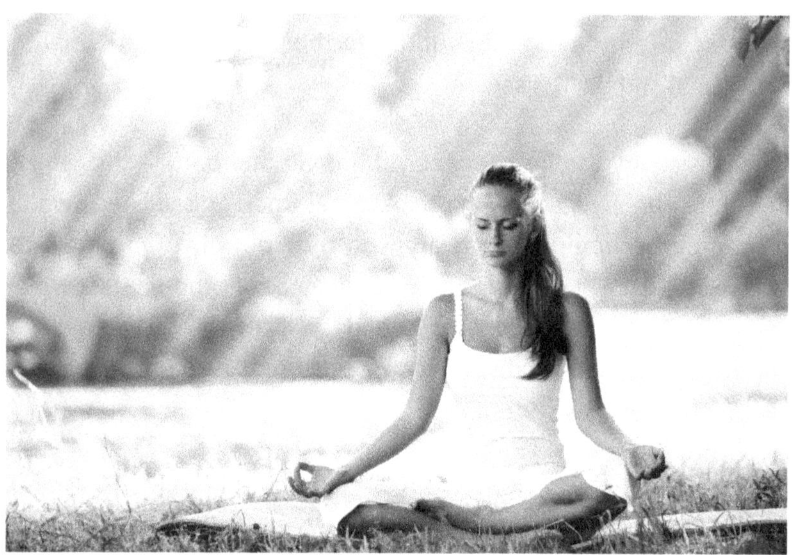

- **For Spiritual Healing**

Everything in life is a contribution of two factors, cause, and effect. In using medications to treat ailments, diseases, or illnesses, only the effect is addressed and not the root cause of the problem in the first place. This then allows for the problem to keep reoccurring and further treatment has to be sought.

It's a vicious cycle that most people today take for granted as the medication often work quickly and satisfactorily to rid the problem. Most main causes of diseases, ailments, and illnesses are because of poor diets, chemicals ingested in the form of medications or the general attitude of the individual.

Yoga techniques address these very important aspects with postures and poses and deep breathing exercises. Besides the yoga regiment of exercises, there is also another side of yoga that one can specifically train on. This is the spiritual side of yoga.

Spiritual yoga teaches the individual how to attain a simple outlook in life and not too busy the mind with always chasing material things with the intention of gaining satisfaction. Yoga teaches how to get in touch with the inner man. Through the poses and meditations, the inner self can become centered and thus create a very powerful energy source which in turn can provide the healing force necessary to heal.

Being able to draw from this inner power should be the goal of every person's spiritual harmony. Yoga brings together physical movements with philosophical thinking which equates the beginnings of spiritual healing. The spiritual healing process works on three levels. The balancing of energies thought the entire being and maintaining the equilibrium in the consciousness are the focal point.

Using yoga to achieve spiritual healing also does work to the overall benefit of the individual in terms of the reactions one has with the outer elements. With the peace and holistic nature of the individual now possess, little can cause negative effects in his or her life.

- **For Emotional Healing**

The emotional well-being of an individual is very important to maintaining good health and a good attitude in life. If a person's emotional health is not at its optimum positive level then all other part of the body start to break down over time. This negative process is so subtle that very few people if any see the connection at all. All emotions are considered sacred, it's how these emotions are handled is where the problem lies.

In the practice of yoga the individual learns how to calm the body and mind and teaches the mind how to reach a level of peace and contentment. When this is successfully understood and learnt then the emotional healing process can take place. Armed with the emotional strength derived from learning yoga the individual learns the difference between responding to a situation or conflict as opposed to reacting to it.

Emotional healing helps the individual develop the thinking that reacting to negative situation, instinctively with emotions like anger, frustration, and grief can be controlled and turned into responding to the situation with a more positive attitude. This then allows the yoga technique to promote emotional healing from within to avoid any outside negative energy from seeping in. in this way the individual gets to stay connected to the spirit and truth of the inner self.

Healing emotionally through the use of yoga ensure the individual no longer looks upon a situation with the view of being victimized, rather this ability now gives the individual the strength to reinforce the self-identity with confidence. On a cellular level even the body cell imprint the corresponding emotions in our thoughts and replicate them in the cell make up. Therefore connecting the healing pattern with the now optimum healing levels brings about both positive elements into the body and mind.

# Chapter 9 - The Right Diet for Optimum Yoga Efficiency

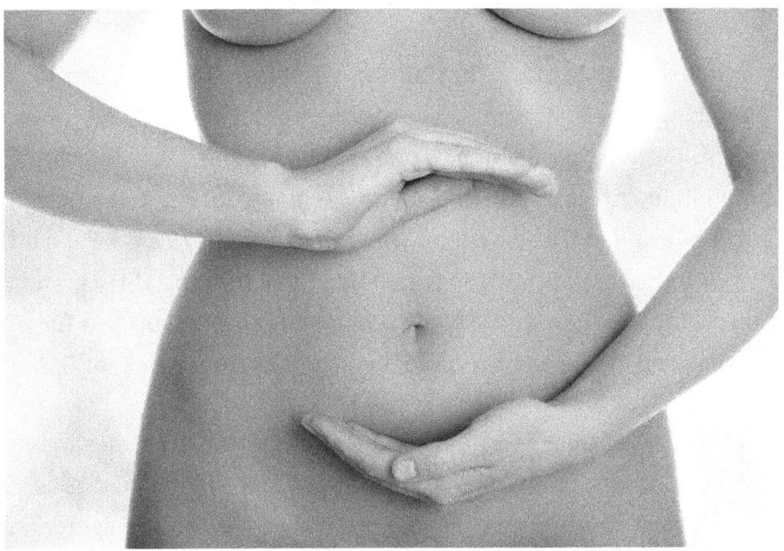

The body needs food for two purposes, as fuel to supply our energy, and to repair body tissues. Four elements are needed for the building of the body and for its repair, namely (1) protein or nitrogenous food, (2) carbohydrates, (3) fats or hydrocarbons, and (4) minerals, these four elements being found in greater proportions in vegetables than in flesh foods. The most valuable vegetable sources of protein are cheese, soya beans, nuts, peas and milk, and the most wholesome sources of starches and sugars are honey, whole wheat, oats, unpolished rice, and potatoes. Fruits and vegetables, as well as supplying organic minerals and hydrocarbons, also aid in keeping an alkaline reserve in the blood, essential for carrying waste carbon dioxide to the lungs for elimination.

I am not going to try to convert any of my meat-eating readers to vegetarianism (as the practice of Yoga will do this for me in time), but I would say this: Although the meat eater may look strong and healthy he has not the endurance, the staying power, and the resistance to disease of the vegetarian. That a natural diet of fruits, greens, milk and dairy products, citrus fruits, and whole grains is man's ideal and vitamin-packed health-giving diet.

It is interesting to note that all food is originally produced in a vegetable form and is in effect stored up sunshine. Think of an orange. The next time you pick one up to peel and eat it and throw the vitamin-rich skin into the dustbin, think of it as it really is, a parcel of distilled sunshine. And why throw the peel away? Eat a bit of it with the rest of the orange and what you do not eat try grating it into various other foods to add a rich and tangy flavor. It is full of vitamins and added to a jar of honey it adds that extra something.

So to eat vegetables is to eat distilled sunshine. To eat flesh is to take vegetable food secondhand from another animal, and here it is interesting to note that man eats mainly the flesh of vegetarian animals such as cows, pigs, sheep, and poultry, deer, and rabbits. He does not eat the flesh of carnivorous animals.

Why kill helpless and friendly animals? Why subject them to the pain and terror of the slaughterhouse when there is so much goodness to eat from the clean earth? Why take a life away when we can eat fruit off the trees, and all the bounty of the harvest? Why all this violence in the name of good eating? Why not have mercy? The pure in mind do not kill, and the pure in body do not need to kill. Think, do think, about it first the next time you cut a piece of steak and carry it on your fork to your mouth; think of the animal that died in pain to provide you with this supper of yours. Are you sure it is worth it? And are fruit and vegetables and nuts not more pleasant to handle than wet and bleeding pieces of a dead animal?

It is interesting to note that once a person becomes a vegetarian and knows the health and purity which results from eating good and pure food, he seldom if ever reverts back to the lower type of food. As he grows spiritually, man ceases to desire flesh foods. Thus man's choice of foods is directly influenced by his degree of mental purity.

And so the Yoga diet is simply to keep as closely as possible to natural foods. This means plenty of nuts, whole cereals, and fresh fruits and juices. From these, man can get all the vitamins, proteins, carbohydrates and minerals he needs. From these also he has the means whereby to nourish the cells of the body without overburdening the system with unnatural and alien foods and drinks. It should be noted that even the most perfect system cannot work to the maximum of its efficiency when it is fed with unnatural foods.

What, then, are these unnatural foods to be avoided? These are the refined, processed, tinned and packaged foods, the worst offenders being white sugar, white flour, white rice and any other food from which the vitality has been refined out. Pickles, preserves, sweets and over-salted foods should be avoided, as should anything containing artificial ingredients. This, 1 know, is not easy if one tends to eat out a great deal. Well-meaning relations and friends hand us heavily iced sweet cakes and sandwiches made with that unwholesome substance, white bread. What can one do to avoid complete social ostracism? That is a problem which you can work out for yourselves, according to your individual circumstances but to all of you I would say this, avoid these foods wherever possible but do not, in the process, offend anyone. Rather eat a piece of cake than hurt someone's feelings. You can leave most of it in crumbs on your plate without arousing suspicion.

The three main rules of the Yoga diet are (1) non-violence, (2) moderation, and (3) attitude of mind. Non-violence I have already discussed. What then of moderation? You must train yourself to eat only what you need and no more. As you proceed with your studies of Yoga you will find yourself taking less interest in food and more interest in spiritual matters. Food no longer becomes a break from the round of work. It becomes a time of refueling the body so that it may continue to flourish. Remember to chew each mouthful slowly which simple practice will gradually accustom you to taking only as much food as you need, not as much as you think you want. By all means enjoy your food but take it in moderation.

And what of attitude of mind? It is not necessary for you to become cranks and food faddists who measure every mouthful you eat. It is not necessary for you to set up a hue and cry about the needless slaughter of animals for food. Quietly pursue your own course, eat only what is pure and natural and your influence will be far greater on those around you than by any more noisy methods.

I am by no means deaf to the many arguments against vegetarianism that are hurled at me from time to time. They go as follows. If everyone became a vegetarian we should be completely overrun by animals. That without eating flesh our diet becomes dull and uninteresting. That the vegetarian diet is not filling and the amount of food one has to consume to satisfy one's hunger tends to make one gain weight. That one becomes socially 'difficult' and eating out becomes something of a problem. That the fancy health food shops are much more expensive than the other food shops. These are the main objections although there are many more. Let us demolish each one in turn.

First, there's the danger of us being overrun by animals if everyone became a vegetarian. Not true, for the simple reason that animals raised for commercial slaughter are artificially bred to multiply at a greater rate than is natural. If it became unprofitable to breed animals the number of them would be drastically decreased by introducing alternate breeding methods.

From the economic standpoint, if everyone became a vegetarian the area of land used to graze animals for food could be used to raise anything from four to forty times as much vegetable food. Meat is actually no more than very expensive, secondhand, vegetable food. It is a known fact that vegetable foods can be produced much more economically than flesh foods.

Let us then consider the second argument against vegetarianism, that the vegetarian diet is dull and uninteresting. To a cook who is imaginative and adventurous, this need not be so. To one who is not, a flesh diet is equally as unpalatable for a good cook can show her talent with any kind of food. And what can be more colorful and exotic than a plate full of mixed and brightly colored vegetables topped with grated cheese. What a conglomeration of colors, textures, and flavors. What a wealth of vitamins, and what easily digestible nourishment. Food without killing - surely that is the ideal diet for a thinking man?

The third argument, that the vegetarian becomes socially a difficult customer, is one which the strong minded will choose to ignore. If your ideals and beliefs are against the killing of innocent animals and the eating of their flesh, then you will not mind being misunderstood by well-meaning friends and relatives. Those closest to you will be only too ready to respect your wishes. As far as eating at restaurants is concerned there are many fine and economical vegetarian restaurants up and down the country and if your own particular district has none you could always take your own packed lunch to work. You can always get round the difficulties if you really want to.

And the fourth argument that the vegetarian diet is not filling enough and that the extra intake of food tends to make one gain weight? What of this? This is where the eating habits of the Yogis will help you. They chew their food slowly and at the same time very gradually decrease their intake of food until they are eating only enough to keep alive and superbly healthy. More food than this amount is superfluous and tends to put on weight but you will notice that no devotee of Yoga has even an ounce of superfluous fat on him or her.

And what of the last argument, I mentioned that health food shops are expensive markets and eat up the household budget? True, if you do not bother to learn vegetarian cookery. If you are a housewife, and your cooking is good and tasty, then perhaps your husband and your children will become vegetarians too. If you live alone you have no one to consider but yourself, and if you are a bachelor, your mother, your sister or even an understanding landlady will come to the rescue. What I am impressing on would-be vegetarians is that it can be done if you really want to. And I am not asking you at this stage to become a vegetarian but merely making various practical suggestions as to how it can be done in the event of your gradually turning against the eating of flesh foods for the reasons I have already outlined.

This is a book about Hatha Yoga and I am writing it mainly from the point of view of your health. However, the body and the mind being inseparable, in showing you how to discipline the one I cannot but mention from time to time the effect upon the other. As Yoga gives your body a new lightness and suppleness you will find that you have gradually become a more spiritual person and food will be of less importance to you than before. You will become more sensitive to the feelings of others and therefore stop to consider the feelings of helpless animals in slaughterhouses up and down the country.

You who long to be slim, to regain your youthful suppleness and vitality, are going to be helped to this end not, as I warned you at the beginning, by any magical or 'crash' diet, but simply by adjusting you're eating habits and way of thinking. Where to begin?

First of all remember that our bodies are only nourished by food which they can break down and assimilate and that, ideally, all food should be laxative. This is far from the case, however, and far too much devitalized and unnatural food is being consumed in this modern world with the result that an appallingly high percentage of the population suffers from constipation and other disorders of the digestive tract. The Yogis name constipation as 'the Mother of all diseases', and here we might aptly name devitalized food as 'the mother of all constipation and digestive disorders'.

What is devitalized food and why are the Yogis so against it? Dead and devitalized foods include everything that has been preserved, bottled, bleached, refined, canned, pickled, or polished. When I say avoid eating white flour products, white sugar products, and polished rice you will ask why. What is wrong with these substances? Simply that in their refined state they are unsuitable as foods and are actually harmful to the human body. What is wrong with eating raw sugar, whole wheat flour products, and unpolished rice? They may prove somewhat dearer but who in his right mind would try to economize on good food? And in the case of raw sugar be careful that you are not buying refined sugar that has simply been colored brown. And try, for a change, to sweeten your food with honey. More easily assimilated than any other food, it is especially beneficial to older people and those of you who are suffering from digestive troubles of any kind.

Being a lifelong honey eater I cannot impress on you too strongly how wholesome and nutritious a food this is. The purest and most natural of foods, it is cheap and plentiful and yet so few people recognize its enormous value.

I seem to hear protests in my ears already. Do you say that you once bought a jar of honey, and you tried to eat it and what happened? It simply would not go down. You dislike the stuff and that is that. But wait. Perhaps you once bought a pound of sour apples. Did you then decide never to buy apples again because you disliked the taste of sour ones? There are very many different honeys. Maybe the jar you once bought was a blended honey, better used in cooking. Why not try one of the dark honeys, brown as a nut, with the strong and heady sweetness of sunshine? Why not try one of the mild, creamy white honeys, thick and subtle flavored? There is such a bewildering variety of honeys from all over the world that I could not possibly name them all, but perhaps the most delectable of all, though it is a matter of personal preference, are the clover honeys, smooth and mellow as butterscotch, and with an unforgettable bouquet, and the dark-toned, exotic honeys of the Caribbean.

And do not, please, think that honey is always clear golden or biscuit colored. Honeys are as multi-colored as a rainbow. The French honey that is gathered from the blooms of gooseberry and sycamore trees is an exquisite sea green. The flavor, need I say, is beyond words. From Brazil comes a black honey, from Africa a clear, pale green, and from Texas comes one of the most unique honeys in the world, the remarkable guajillo honey which is crystal white with a pearly reflection like new milk. Not always available in American "health-food" stores, but to be looked for at any rate, is the exotic lotus honey of India. It is as exciting, as mysterious, and as health giving as Yoga itself. I could go on for whole book writing ecstatically of the wonder and the glories of honey but let it suffice to say that if you think you dislike honey then try all the different ones you can find. If you fail to find one you like you are indeed unique.

If you feel I was becoming lyrical over honey I am going to be just the opposite about its greatest rival—sugar. Why, I wonder, did we abandon honey, nature's most nutritious sweet food, in favor of dry, sterile, refined sugars? I am afraid that there can be only one answer—sheer ignorance of the basic needs and capabilities of the human organism. Because, up to about the year 1700 sugar was the exclusive amenity of the aristocracy, it came to be greatly prized by the masses as a delicacy. It had a certain social significance as, say, caviar has today. So when a new process was discovered of refining sugar cheaply and in large quantities honey began to lose its popularity as a sweetening agent and became increasingly less available as sugar became more so.

Then physicians in America and Europe began to realize that a tragic dietary mistake was being made and that the over indulgence in artificial sugars was causing increasing ill health. New digestive and nervous disorders began to make their appearance, and the instance of diabetes shot up alarmingly.

Many people do not know that granulated sugars, syrups, treacle, and molasses are artificial sweets. Still fewer people know that they are also powerful stimulants, drugs which are actually habit forming. So used are people to taking them as an everyday commodity that they have come to regard them as harmless, pleasant, and nourishing. I assure you that they are neither harmless nor nourishing though no doubt many would protest that they are pleasant.

The sweets that 1 have mentioned are manufactured by a process which destroys all their nutritive elements. In the case of granulated sugar the sugar crystals that are formed after the cane juice is treated with the fumes of burning sulphur or heated with bisulphide of lime, are sterile and devitalized. It is just this fact which makes sugar a commodity that will keep almost indefinitely which is a distinct advantage from a commercial point of view but hardly from a health one.

Sugar granules, in their final, highly concentrated form, are powerful stimulants. When they reach the human stomach they oxidize violently upon their contact with oxygen, which produces an explosive effect upon the digestive system and causes an increased activity in the internal organs. White sugar can be compared with a highly combustible fuel that violently ignites, burns with a fierce intensity, and as quickly dies down.

Can you imagine the shock treatment all this activity has on the digestive and nervous systems? And because of this fast dying down the body is aware of a hunger for more and more sugar. It is this fact that makes people often eat as much as a pound of sweets or chocolates at one sitting. The desire for 'just one more' becomes a compulsion, and the more poorly nourished a person is the more susceptible he will be to sugar addiction. For that is what it is, an addiction, no less. That sugar, in the last analysis, can cause serious malnutrition is proved by the fact that although like alcohol, it is a quick source of energy the effects do not last and as the body becomes more and more dependent on these 'quick lifts' it becomes less inclined to eat nourishing food.

To sum up the case for honey and the case against sugar I would say this. Those artificial sugars must be broken down by the digestive tract into simple sugars before they can be utilized by the body, and thus they put an undue strain upon the system. The use of honey presents no such problems as it consists entirely of natural sugars that do not have to be oxidized by the digestive tract. Honey is absorbed at once without excessive stimulation or shock to the system and it does not result in a craving for more. Sugar is no substitute for honey as, chemically, it is of an entirely different nature. So why be dictated to by the heavy hand of commerce?

In order to guide you in your choice of foods for your Yoga diet I will here outline the principle vitamins and their easily available food sources. Vitamins, in controlling the body's use of minerals, promote a balance in the body necessary for the proper functioning of the endocrine glands and the formation of hormones.

Vitamin A

The body uses this vitamin best in conjunction with vitamin D in the proportion of 7-1. The principle sources of vitamin A are cabbage, carrots, celery, endive, lettuce, oranges, parsley, prunes and dried apricots, spinach, tomatoes, and watercress.

Lack of vitamin A produces scaly skin, stones in the kidney and gall bladder, catarrh and sinus infections, poor digestion, and low resistance to disease. This vitamin is essential for proper growth of body tissues, and increases resistance to infections of the urinary and respiratory tracts.

**Vitamin Bx**

The principle sources are cabbage, carrots, celery, coconuts, citrus fruits, parsley, radishes, turnip tops, and watercress.

A lack of vitamin B1 results in low heartbeats, poor appetite, gastric, intestinal and nervous disorders, chronic constipation and the enlargement of the adrenal glands and the pancreas. Violent exercise, increasing age and weight, and feverishness all increase the body's need for this vitamin.

**Vitamin B2**

The main sources are apples, apricots, cabbage, carrots, coconuts, citrus fruits, prunes, spinach, turnip tops, and watercress. The supply of this vitamin decreases when there are an increase in the consumption of fats and minerals, and are conserved by the intake of fibrous foods.

If there isn't enough vitamin B2, there will be low energy and stamina, loss of hair, cataract and tongue ulceration as well as disorders of the digestive tract.

**Vitamin C**

I would mention that copper cooking vessels cause a serious loss of this vitamin. The main sources of it are citrus fruits, cucumber, parsley, pineapples, radishes, rhubarb, tomatoes, turnips, watercress, carrots, and green leafy vegetables.

Lack of this vitamin causes many illnesses, among them being weakness and shortness of breath, palpitations, headaches, tooth decay, peptic and duodenal ulcers; heart disease, circulatory disease, and the impaired function of the adrenal glands.

**Vitamin D**

This vitamin is stored in the skin as ergosterol, which is converted into vitamin D2 by sunshine or ultra-violet light. Vitamin D controls the calcium content in the blood; excess of vitamin D results in a number of disorders, including diarrhea, depression, and severe toxic disturbances.

Lack of this vitamin means fragile bones, rickets and bow legs, poor retention, and cramps resulting from abnormally low calcium metabolism. Though this vitamin is not found in fruits, vegetables and cereals, butter is an excellent source as is cod liver oil, for non-vegetarians. For the vegetarians there are a number of artificial sources of vitamin D, among them irradiated ergosterol.

**Vitamin E**

This vitamin is stored in the muscles and fat and as it is rapidly depleted it must be renewed regularly. The main sources of it are wheat germ, celery, lettuce, leafy green vegetables, and parsley. According to recent medical research, lack of vitamin E can produce sterility in sexes, miscarriage, and loss of hair.

**Minerals**

The following minerals have been declared essential to the human body by research authorities—calcium, chlorine, copper, iodine, iron, magnesium, manganese, phosphorus, potassium, sodium, and sulphur. I will describe each one briefly, listing the main food sources.

Calcium (alkaline). Daily requirements, adults 10 grains, children 15 grains. This mineral builds strong bones and teeth, aids heart action and the clotting of the blood, and helps to establish the correct balance of vitamin D in the body.

Main sources of calcium are cheese, milk, citrus fruits, green leafy vegetables, carrots, celery, figs, rhubarb, and parsley. Blackberries and cranberries are also a good source of this mineral.

Chlorine. This is a general cleanser of the body and helps to expel waste matter and purify the blood. It also aids in the formation of gastric and other digestive juices. The main sources of this mineral are fruits and vegetables.

Copper (acid forming). The main sources of this mineral, which are necessary for the absorption of iron in the body, are leafy vegetables as well as fresh and dried fruits.

Iodine (acid forming). As this mineral is essential to the proper functioning of the thyroid gland, deficiency in it results in goitre and general glandular disturbances. The main sources of it are green leafy vegetables, carrots, cucumber, prunes, radishes, pineapples, and tomatoes.

Iron (alkaline). This is the mineral that figures prominently in the building of red corpuscles, and which also absorbs and carries oxygen in the bloodstream to all parts of the body. There must be adequate supplies of chlorophyll and copper in the diet to effect the proper assimilation of iron, and some experts consider that a woman needs three to four times as much as a man. The main sources of iron are whole wheat, oatmeal, dried beans, dried peas and dried fruits, green leafy vegetables, cheese, tomatoes, bananas, and fresh string beans. Lack of iron results in anemia and general fatigue.

Magnesium (alkaline). This is the mineral that keeps teeth and bones strong and hard. It also helps to build cells, particularly of the lungs and nerves, and also helps to form albumin in the blood. Insufficiency of these minerals results in poor blood circulation, constipation, and acidity. The main sources of this mineral are nuts, whole wheat, unpolished rice, oatmeal, dried fruits, and leafy vegetables.

Phosphorus (acid forming). This is another mineral essential to the building of sound bones and teeth and it also maintains the alkalinity of the bloodstream by the phosphates it forms. The most important sources of this mineral are nuts, particularly almonds, cereals, grapes, citrus fruits, blackberries and cranberries, cucumbers, whole wheat, wheat germ, soya beans, tomatoes, and watermelons.

Potassium (alkaline). This is the mineral basis of all muscular tissue, and is vital to the correct functioning of the liver. The main sources of this mineral are leafy green vegetables, fruits and nuts.

Sodium (alkaline). Though this mineral is important to the" body in forming the digestive juices, the saliva, bile, and pancreatic juices, and for the elimination of carbon dioxide, table salt is not the most beneficial source. It is far better to obtain it from its natural sources such as whole wheat, rye bread, buttermilk, celery, bananas, leafy vegetables, and beetroot.

Sulphur (acid forming). This mineral has an antiseptic effect on the alimentary canal, is a constituent of the hemoglobin and keeps the blood purified, and prevents toxic impurities from accumulating in the body. All fruits and vegetables are good sources of sulphur but these should be well balanced with foods of high phosphorus content such as milk, cheese and eggs, cereals and nuts. Foods high in phosphorus but low in sulphur can lead to improper balance of these minerals in the body.

The above will serve as a useful guide to your future eating habits and with a little experimenting you will find a diet that keeps you healthy and provides all the essential elements you need. Though diet is very much a matter of individual taste and circumstances, here is a list of 'musts' that I learned from my own Yoga teacher.

If you do not want anything, then do not eat it even if you think it is good for you. By all means eat meat if you like it but do not eat it merely because you think you cannot live without it. Apart from cheese, eggs, and nuts, the soya bean products, weight for weight, contain more protein than the best steak. Soya bean is not only cheaper and more nutritious but it is also non-acid forming. Eat a little less of everything but do effect this very gradually.

Do not starve yourself or suffer hunger pains between meals but do try to cut down on your intake of food. Avoid the 'dead' and devitalized foods, i.e. everything refined, bleached, or preserved. Eat whole wheat bread, raw sugar, or honey. When eating fruit, do not throw away the peel. Eat it with the fruit, or in the case of oranges, lemons, or tangerines the peel can be grated to add a delicious and tangy flavor to other foods.

Always cook potatoes in their jackets, either baked or boiled. Much of the protein in potatoes is usually thrown away with the peel. And remember the tops of celery, carrots, turnips and beetroots are too nutritious to be thrown away. Cut them up and steam them with the rest of your vegetables. Instead of serving just one vegetable at a meal, cut up several kinds and steam them very slowly in very little water. Do not overcook; in fact many vegetarians prefer chopped or diced vegetables to be slightly underdone. This preserves the natural texture and flavor.

Always cook vegetables slowly in a pan with a tight fitting lid and avoid copper cooking pans if possible. Do not drink too much tea or coffee as tannic acid and caffeine are not beneficial to the body. By all means enjoy a cup of tea or coffee but make a mental note that you will gradually cut down your intake. At the same time try to drink more milk, either hot or cold, but please never iced. Do not throw away water in which vegetables have been cooked. Why dump vitamins down the sink when they make an excellent basis for soups? With a little seasoning added they are very palatable to drink just as they are.

Avoid fried foods especially if you are over forty. When you do eat fatty foods choose what are known as unsaturated fats—corn oil, sunflower seed oil, and soya bean oil. Avoid animal fats such as butter, lard, and dripping, and also avoid olive oil and margarine. Experiment with cheeses. They are all a wonderful source of protein and America alone has many fine cheeses with which to vary your diet to say nothing of the delicious cheeses from other countries.

Be adventurous, try new things, and above all eat only what is pure and natural. Do not over-indulge and whenever you are tempted to reach for that chocolate box go to the fruit bowl or the honey pot instead. Try dates instead of sweets. To conclude I will list the five basic Yoga rules for the maintenance of health and the prevention of disease. Eat natural wholesome food, enough and no more for the body's needs.

Proper breathing and breath control exercises, for the increased oxygenation of the blood. Regular exercises stimulate the circulation and to keep the spine supple and healthy. The practice of concentration and meditation, and the correct method of directing the thoughts towards the positive encourage spiritual growth.

# Chapter 10 - Is Yoga the Answer to Female Disorders?

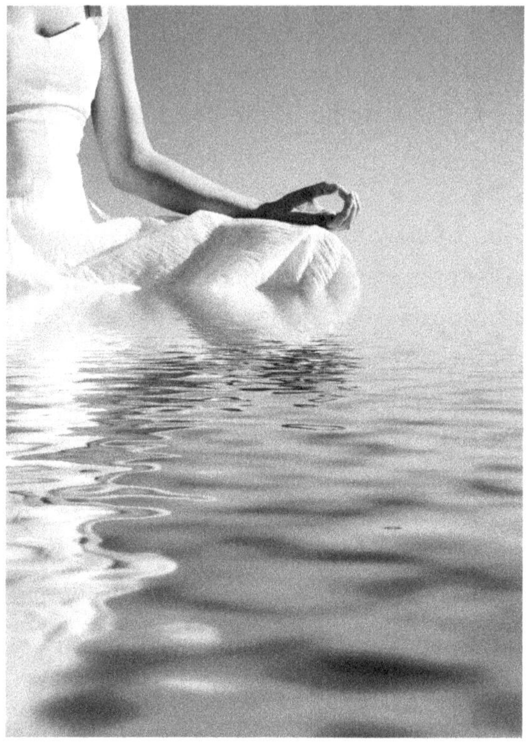

If half the female Yoga enthusiasts I know began their study of Hatha Yoga for the sake of improving their figures, it can be safely said that the other half did so because of menstrual pains and other female disorders. Many females find that drugs do little to alleviate the dragging down pains they have to endure every month, and so year after year they suffer in silence.

But this kind of pain is unnecessary. Yoga can and does help. Practice, at least twice a day throughout the month, the Sarvangasana or Shoulder stand, or if you are unable to do this, try lying down with your feet very much higher than your head. The chief function of this inverted posture in the battle against period pains lies in the reversal of the influence of gravity upon the internal organs. The fluids of the body tend naturally to flow downwards and even the skeleton is subject to downward displacement by the pull of gravity. The downward drag, though it may be held in check by a healthy and active body, is nevertheless always present in some degree.

There is a greater tendency in women than in men to suffer from varicose veins and prolapse of the viscera, this being due to the wider pelvis and larger number of abdominal organs. By inverting the body and holding it in poised stillness, all downward pressure is relieved. Practice the Shoulder stand over a period of time and you will soon begin to notice a lessening of the intensity of your discomfort each month, until after a time it will cease altogether to be a problem. Though a certain degree of slowing down of activity on the first two days of a period is advisable, there need not be any undue resting. Incidentally the Shoulder stand is especially recommended for women after childbirth after a suitable period of recuperation has elapsed, but in all cases do not prolong the posture beyond the point of absolute comfort. No Yoga exercises should be performed during pregnancy or menstruation except the breathing ones, which can be done with impunity.

An especially valuable exercise for women suffering from ovarian and uterine disorders is the BHUJANGASANA, called in English the COBRA POSE. AS it belongs to the basic group of essential Yoga asanas it should never be omitted from any practice schedule, no matter what the ailment from which you are suffering. It is not at all difficult and can be performed by beginners in all age groups.

**Cobra Pose**

Lie face downwards on your mat with your chin on the ground, and your legs straight and feet together. Place your palms on the floor at shoulder level keeping your elbows high off the ground. Inhale slowly and deeply and at the same time slowly raise your head, shoulders, chest and upper abdomen, leaving the lower part of your abdomen on the floor.

Keep arching your spine as you complete your inhalation, and remain thus for as long as you comfortably can without exhaling. You will feel a strong pressure in the lower part of your back as you push your head back as far as you can. And remember to keep your elbows bent and well off the floor.

When the impulse to exhale appears, do so and at the same time gradually lower your body until you are once more touching the floor with your chin. Without pausing, inhale again and repeat the movement and after the second performance of the Cobra relax before you repeat the exercise a third and fourth time.

The Cobra has many benefits and is as suitable for men as for women for it affects the adrenal glands which lie above each kidney, and the backward bend of the Cobra sends them a richer supply of blood and subjects them to a healthy pressure. The Cobra is also beneficial to people suffering from backache, displaced vertebrae, and poor circulation.

A word of warning though, you may not be used to exercising and your spine may be stiffer than you think so do please be careful while bending backwards in this exercise. Be sure not to jerk your body as you raise it off the ground as you could easily injure a rigid muscle and the pain could last some time. Remember that the Cobra is a beautiful and graceful exercise. As you leave the floor come up slowly and majestically like a rising cobra and under no circumstances must you force yourself to hold the position longer than you find comfortable. Gradually increase the time you hold it until you can remain immobile in the Cobra pose for ten seconds.

When you are limbered up you can perform this asana up to six times a day.

While the Cobra is particularly useful to women suffering from dysmenorrhea, amenorrhea, leucorrhea, and various other utero-ovaries troubles, the overall benefits can be greatly increased by those students able to increase the backward bend. Do not perform the variation until you are able to do the Cobra I have just described with perfect ease and comfort.

**Cobra**

Variation 2. From the first position, rise into the Cobra with the elbows bent and the spine arched. Slowly straighten the elbows, push the head back as far as you can, so that the bending of the spine involves the sacral to the cervical region. Remain thus for as long as you comfortably can without strain and then relax. When you can perform variation 2 you can, if you wish, omit variation 1 from your practice schedule.

Variation 3. There is yet a third variation of the lovely Cobra Pose for advanced students but it can be achieved by beginners who are athletic or who have been trained in ballet. From variation 2, with elbows straight, bend the spine backwards still farther; gradually bring your toes towards your head to touch the back of your head. This tones the deep and the superficial muscles of the back, and also relieves backache, helping to keep the spine young and supple.

And now to return to another inverted posture to rest the internal organs. For my readers who find the Shoulder stand just a little too strenuous but who need the benefits of this valuable posture, there is a slightly easier posture which has the delightful name of VIPARITA-KARANI MUDRA, meaning literally reverse effect. For short we will call it THE REVERSE POSE.

The radiations which we receive from the earth are negative while those from the cosmos are positive. Thus, when in the ordinary standing position we receive the negative radiation through the soles of our feet and the positive radiation through the top of the skull. In the Yoga poses in which the body is turned upside down, viz. Shoulder stand, Headstand, and Reverse Pose, the effect is just the opposite. Additionally these postures bring an unaccustomed rich supply of blood to the lower intestinal organs.

# About the Author

Aileen Gomez is a yoga instructor. She came from Mexico and is living in the US for only three years after she married and American.

Aileen first became a yoga enthusiast when she was introduced to it during a trip to India. She became fascinated with the art that she learned as much as she can and repeated the knowledge at home.

Today, Aileen is an expectant mother.